MW00745243

CARING FOR

THE CAREGIVER

CARING FOR
THE CAREGIVER

A SPIRITUAL APPROACH
FOR THE PROFESSIONAL

Kathleen J. Rusnak, Ph.D.

THE BRICK WALL 2, INC.

Caring for the Caregiver:
A Spiritual Approach for the Professional
by Kathleen J. Rusnak, Ph.D.

Published by:
The Brick Wall 2, Inc.
21 Mohawk Trail, PBN 263
Greenfield, Massachusetts 01301
www.thebrickwall2.com
(413) 446-8653

For information on bulk purchase of this book, contact
the publisher at thebrickwall2@aol.com

ISBN: 978-0-615-27805-6

Design and composition: www.dmargulis.com

MANUFACTURED IN THE UNITED STATES OF AMERICA

DEDICATION

To all those called *to be caregivers*

CONTENTS

PREFACE

COMMENTS I've received from caregivers who have heard my lecture on this subject compelled me to write this essay. They express the relief of caregivers to finally be the topic of a lecture. "No one ever asks how I am," one man commented to me afterward, "They only ask how my wife is doing." Another said, "You name exactly what I have been going through. I didn't know anyone else felt like me." Another comment was most telling: "I never considered myself a caregiver. I didn't even know there was a word for what I do, a caregiver. I only thought of myself as his wife." Another person said, "Thank you for telling me the spiritual path I am on and the importance of what I am doing."

When I give this lecture as part of an online course for professional caregivers, they too express their own lack of awareness of the spiritual journey that caregivers are thrown into. They are moved by the metaphors that name various dimensions of their journey; and they acknowledge their own need to be aware of them in order to care for the caregivers with empathy, compassion, and support.

While the lecture was originally given for caregivers, this book is intended for professional staff and for family members, neighbors, or friends who care for the caregivers. The focus of this essay is the unique journey of caregivers caring for persons with dementia. Although this type of care calls for unprecedented skill and creativity on the part of caregivers, the reality is that all those who are caregivers for persons with life threatening or chronic illnesses will venture on a spiritual journey that takes them through changes they did not anticipate or ask for. This book is for them too.

CARING FOR
THE CAREGIVER

INTRODUCTION

CAREGIVERS—those who attend to
the needs of persons with life threatening or chronic illnesses—venture on a
spiritual journey that takes them through
changes they did not anticipate or ask for.
This book is for professional staff whose
unit of care includes the caregiver and the
patient, as well as for family members,
neighbors, and friends of caregivers. It
can also provide insight to caregivers
themselves.

The content is arranged pasto-
rally; the structure frames the caregivers'

story from their perspective, illuminat-
ing their humanness, frailty, fears, and
hopes. It is *not* intended to give information only. There is no outline of points to
learn. This isn't a cookbook of how-tos
or stages. Rather, I share with you the
approach I use to enter into the caregivers' world, to travel with them into a
place they know well but don't know
that others know about. This approach
includes humor that takes the caregiver
to a mostly unconscious and honest place
within themselves; empathy in naming,
describing, and normalizing their feelings, struggles, confusion, and joys; and
hope in offering new ways of seeing,
coping, and moving forward. Finally, it
offers a deep affirmation of who caregivers are and what they do, along with the
possibility of meaning, beyond the per-

formance of the immediate tasks, of the
inner journey they find themselves on.

This book may look like it is for
the non-professional caregiver of a loved
one at home. But it is designed to aid
those of us who care for caregivers, to let
us know their world (how we might enter
into it) and to describe the possible spiritual places caregivers may travel in this
new role. My goal with this book is to aid
you in supporting caregivers.

I suggest that this kind of structure is a pastoral or spiritual structure in
that it encompasses and invites what the
late Jewish philosopher, Martin Buber
calls an "I–Thou" relationship between
the caregiver and the one being cared
for. "I–Thou" is in contrast to "I–It," in
which the other person is treated as an
object and not as a person. In "I–Thou"

interactions, there is equality within the relationship, and each person's humanity is respected and honored.

In our relationship with caregivers, we try to enter into an "I–Thou" relationship with the caregiver. Such a relationship can preempt, or at least make understandable, the anger and projection that flow from the caregiver to professional staff or friends of a caregiver.

This is but a brief look into one approach and understanding of caregivers. I do not pretend to cover every issue or possibility in this book, but I hope to open the door to deeper thinking, understanding, intentionality, and relationship within those of us who care for caregivers.

SETTING THE STAGE:
THE OPENING

W H E N I'm speaking to caregivers
of persons with dementia, I often begin
with this question: When you were a
child, how many of you said "when I
grow up I want to be a caregiver?" The
raucous laughter that follows is obvi-
ously an expression of relief—relief that
sets the foundation for the rest of the
lecture. They can now let their guard
down, be relaxed. They slouch a bit in
their seats, and their shoulders loosen up.

They no longer have to pretend with me
or deny to themselves or each other that
caring for their loved one with dementia
is something they are enthusiastic about
doing or feel comfortable doing. They are
relieved that they are not going to hear
more unrealistic demands on their already
full plates. They have laughed together at
themselves and at each other. The audience is connected with each other. The
audience is connected with me. They feel
understood, their personhood kindly and
honestly regarded. A trust is born.

R ELUCTANT
W E S ERVE

L ET ' S acknowledge the *reluctant
caregiver* and then let's look at the issues
underlying the reluctance. The issues are
many, but the most common are feelings
of *inadequacy* to be a caregiver; *resentfulness*
that their lives have changed; *grief* for the
life they no longer have; and, for those
who believe in God, *anger at God* that
they were chosen for the task.

     I begin, as you'll see in a moment,
by identifying their call to be caregivers

as synonymous with the call from God experienced by many of the biblical prophets in the Hebrew scriptures (those brought up in Judaism, Christianity, or Islam can identify), who were reluctant to be prophets but nevertheless followed the call. Religious or not, caregivers get it. I then add another figure, a reluctant hero, from a secular movie. Whether they are into movies or not, they get it. They feel included.

In theology, it is a common to refer to some of the prophets as reluctant prophets. *Individuals did not chose to be prophets; they were called, even torn from their ordinary lives to warn, bless, call to repentance, uplift and reprove, and, at the core of all of their endeavors, to be messengers of hope. According to Jewish philosopher, theologian, and educator Abraham Heschel, "To be a prophet is both a distinction and an affliction." For me to refer to caregivers as* reluctant caregivers *is to extend the reluctance, distinction, and affliction to their service.*

The examples are telling. The Hebrew prophet Jeremiah is called, but he is only a boy. He has a future of what he wants to be in his own mind. He has his whole life ahead of him. He doesn't want to heed the call. "I am only a boy," he says, "I am too young. I have other plans, dreams, visions! Not me!"

Moses is called, but he doesn't feel equal to the job. In fact, he has a speech impediment. He stutters. He stutters when he talks to God to remind him about his stuttering problem and asks God to find someone who can speak better than he can.

And then there is Jonah. Jonah is asked to do the impossible, to go to Ninevah (modern day Baghdad), to the people who destroyed northern Israel (where Jonah is from) and to tell them to repent or be destroyed. Jonah doesn't want them to repent. He wants them destroyed. His answer to God? He simply runs away. After Jonah is swallowed by a great fish and thrown up on a beach, God tells him a second time to go; and he does, but he is never ever happy about it. Never!

You've heard of Frodo, the little Halfling in the movie "Lord of the Rings?" No one ever heard of Jeremiah, Moses, or Jonah either, until they became famous. Frodo and the others are just like you and me, the seemingly unexceptional, the seemingly inadequate—so much so that we wonder why someone better prepared or with more courage and inner strength isn't called in our place. Finally, one day, Frodo says to Gandalf the Wizard, "I wish the ring had never come to me. I wish none of this had happened." And that's our sentiment too.

Yet God, and Gandalf, respond, "So do all who live to see such times, but that is not for them to decide. All we have to decide is what to do with the time that is given to us."

Prophets and caregivers are different, yes, but the same, in that each is called to do something very difficult, called to do something they are not trained for, and called to do something not of their own choosing. But caregivers have a few things over the prophets of old: they have caregiver conferences and caregiver support groups. Prophets didn't have conferences or support! My audiences usually laugh at this. They see they belong to a select group, and maybe even have it a little better. They get the parallel and they feel understood, but they still don't know what is important about being a caregiver. In their minds being a caregiver is just a very regular or ordinary thing.

Reluctance does not necessarily mean that they do not want to take care of their loved one, but that they have hidden feelings that society, friends, and other family members do not allow them to express as part of being a caregiver and that they are uncomfortable admitting to themselves.

The spirituality of it is just beginning to unfold.

SPIRITUAL SHIFT

T H E realization of a *before* and *after* can signify a spiritual shift in the caregiver. Usually this sentiment is expressed in the words, "It feels like I hit a brick wall." This brick wall is a metaphor for the instant of transition from the world *before* to the world *after*.

> *A woman sat with her daughter in front of the doctor, to hear the results of her mini mental status test. The doctor looked at the daughter and then the mother. "I'm afraid you have probable Alzheimer's," the doctor said. The mother's*

head immediately snapped in the direction of her daughter, and she cried out, "Oh, I'm going to miss you!" What this woman knew in that instant was a whole life change. From that moment on, nothing would ever be the same. The script of life had been interrupted.

While the diagnosis of dementia is not a prognosis of six months or less to live, it signifies a change in the expected future. "From that moment on," the daughter told me, "both my mother and I thought differently about life. We began to ask questions we hadn't asked before. Why is this happening to us? What does it mean? What is important? What isn't as we move forward? How will this change our lives in a deeper way?" My own mother asked different questions. She asked what was important to do now. How would she be remembered? What could she do now before it was too late? What was her purpose in life now.

These kinds of questions are existential or spiritual questions. They are usually prompted by a crisis—what I have called a brick wall event—and signify a shift in perspective. We need to let caregivers know that they have hit a brick wall, an immovable object, and they have bounced off it into a world of change, grief, vulnerability, and confusion, in a direction that ultimately may result in a new identity.

The metaphor of hitting a brick wall is powerful. Like all metaphors, it expresses in symbolic language the depth of raw feeling and emotion that cannot be directly expressed in words. Symbolic language emerges only in a context. For instance, only if I have fallen in love and lost that love, will the expression "my heart is broken" emerge as a way of communicating the impact of how the loss affects me. No one in our culture would mistake this phrase as literal, and everyone understands it.

Those of us who have not received a terminal prognosis probably cannot guess at the metaphor expressed by so many, because it is a language that emerges only with life-altering events, and only because its reality, like a shattered love affair, cannot be expressed in any other way. The realization that follows a brick wall event, "nothing will ever be the same again," is also new to the caregiver. For many, it is the first time they are caring for someone they love who is seriously ill; as a result, so much is new. Perhaps we can understand the shattering impact of their experience by thinking of our own experience of September 11, 2001.

After September 11, we heard over and over that life would never be the same again, that life was forever changed. *And each day changes have happened, ones we never could have anticipated since they seem so distant from the original tragedy. Who would have suspected that car sales would dramatically decrease after September 11, prompting the ripple effect of autoworker layoffs? Who would have imagined a decrease in divorces immediately following September 11? But that is what happened in Texas. Hundreds of other examples could be cited, illustrating that we cannot know what it means when we say that life will be forever changed. We only know that a new reality will continue to unfold for us as the days, weeks, months, and years go by, because we do know one sure thing, that we cannot go back to life as it was before September 11. This is true for our caregivers too.*

No More

ALL change includes loss. Brides and grooms often get cold feet before they take their vows not because, as many suspect, they are unsure of their love for one another, but because in choosing *only* each other, they have inadvertently chosen to close off other relationship options *forever* and to end life in the single world, an entirely different world than the married one.

It would help people immensely who mistake their sadness prior to wedding ceremonies for doubt about their

feelings of love to know that what they
are feeling is grief for the losses that will
accompany the moment of transition, the
change from being single to being married. That moment is one of extreme joy
and a moment of permanent *no mores*.
No more being responsible for only me.
No more playing the field. No more
independent decision-making. No more
single-mindedness. *No more single future!*
Marriage signals a new kind of freedom
for many brides and grooms, but it also
signals the end of freedom as they have
known and experienced it. The end of
single freedom is socially acknowledged
in the ritual of the bachelor parties that
precede weddings, but I wonder how
many people understand that this last
fling is also a grief party.

    Many people do not know that
what they are experiencing is grief or

know that their situation involves grief.
Our society still doesn't acknowledge
the importance of grieving. We hear the
words of Elisabeth Kübler-Ross—that
grief is indicated by shock, denial, anger,
bargaining, and finally by acceptance. But
these are just words. We don't identify
our experiences with these words.

> *Grief means* no more. *I was first introduced to
> this definition by Father Charlie Hudson, the
> founder of The Center For Hope Hospice and
> Palliative Care, in Scotch Plains, New Jersey.
> I have studied grief and read many good books
> on the subject, yet no more stood out as the pri-
> mary practical consequence of loss. As the person
> with dementia declines in memory and function,
> it means no more of whatever the caregiver and
> the person with dementia did together. Maybe
> it means no more travel, no more eating out, no
> more driving, no more conversations, no more
> laughing together.*

Grief is also about one's self, not about the loss of the other person. It is about the "I" who no longer has. In this sense, grief is about "what I have lost" and "what I no longer have" in my life. It is about the holes, gaps, and emptiness that are now recognizable and and that are felt with the absence of what filled its place. Grief is a natural physical, emotional, and spiritual reality.

At a conference, a caregiver approached me expressing terrible feelings of guilt. Her husband had lost his ability to dance, and dancing was something that they both did together at least once a week. "I had a dream a few weeks ago," she said, "In the dream I was dancing with another man and I felt so good. Was I being unfaithful to my husband?" I told her the dream was probably about the loss of her husband's ability to dance the way they used to and not about infidelity. In her dream she compensated for that loss by dancing with someone who could. She felt relieved.

Naming and acknowledging loss for the caregiver helps the caregiver know what they are experiencing and shows deep interest in their situation. The losses are huge and often not recognized by others or given any significance. The losses amount to a slow stripping away—the piling up of *no mores*—that can leave a caregiver vulnerable. The caregiver once had dreams. No more. The caregiver had ideas and beliefs about life and how it should be—a spiritual *no more*. The caregiver lived a certain lifestyle. No more. The caregiver was independent. No more. The caregiver had a companion, a friend, a lover. No more. The caregiver and spouse had a social network. No more. The caregiver had a self-image. No more. The caregiver always had an identity. No more.

Loss is also spiritual in nature. Loss opens a gap that can affect one's faith, positively or negatively. After September 11, 2001, *Frontline* presented "Faith and Doubt at Ground Zero." In this documentary about a Catholic priest, an Episcopal priest, a rabbi, firemen, policemen, and other ordinary citizens directly affected by the terrorism, we heard how trauma and loss affected their beliefs about life. Loss can prompt a person to ask deep existential or spiritual questions: Why did God let this happen to me or my loved one? What does this mean for my life? Who am I now?

Caregivers experience myriad losses. They need to know that their questions, misgivings, and new doubts about beliefs they previously held are normal when the foundation of life is disturbed. Loss can also deepen the foundation upon

which some people stand. Loss can alter,
deepen, or shatter the spiritual self. The
help a caregiver receives from us can
influence which of those the caregiver
experiences.

THE WILDERNESS

WHAT happens to our identity when our world slowly gets stripped away, when the *no mores* leave us empty? "I don't know who I am anymore," one caregiver said to me. He then went on to list all of the losses that had once made up his identity. He said he felt lost and confused.

When someone asks you who you are, how do you identify yourself? Generally, people respond with their name, job, marital status, how many children they have, and sometimes their religion. Our résumés offer more detail—our education, employment past and present, what we have published, organizations we served with, and so on. Some of us walk around with our identities: the medical white jacket, a stethoscope around the neck, collars on clergy, and other indicators that announce our occupations. Other details that signify our status, and thus our identity, include where we live, the kind of car we drive, where we eat, and who we associate with.

We don't often ask ourselves the question, Who am I? We think we already know, until our losses chip away at our exterior world; and then the answer is usually expressed in the negative: "I used to . . ." or "we used to . . . ." Like an onion whose layers are peeled away, our identity, mostly defined by our outer selves, our academic degrees, our accomplishments, our associations, and our roles in life, is called into question.

Carl Jung referred to this aspect of life as "life's morning," when people focus on acquiring the outer expectations of life, the cultural script society writes for us. For too many people, the lure of culture's script is the extent of their development. The second half of life is to retire, enjoy your grandchildren, travel, and finally do what you always wanted to do. A death, a divorce, and other tragedies can force growth, although they can also just make people more depressed and bitter. What matters is the type and quality of help they get. This is true for caregivers, as well.

Jung called the development of the inner life, "life's afternoon." The one-sidedness of life's morning gives way to the possibility of developing the spiritual side of the psyche. On occasion we hear of individuals who have endured what we call a mid-life crisis. We see the husband leave his wife for a younger woman, only to want to return to her later. But it is too late. Or we hear about the person who at forty-five enters medical school or seminary. The stories are powerful and inspiring. A mid-level manager finally gets fed up with the rat race and moves to the mountains. There is a shift from outer world to inner world—from acquisition to meaning-making and meaningful living.

It isn't often that we see this take place. Becoming the person we have the ability to become doesn't just happen. While people who are dying are the best indicators of this reality—often living the script to the hilt, and at life's end, wishing they had lived otherwise—caregivers face this too. Their losses leave them feeling isolated, abandoned. Caregivers discover all too often that everything they held on to in their life, those things that defined who they were, slowly slip away.

When I attended an International Death and Dying Conference in New York City in the 1990s, I asked a Buddhist monk, who was leading one of the workshops, a question about "holding on." He was speaking about the Buddhist belief that suffering is caused by attachment, and later on he made a comment about married monks. I wondered how one could be detached and be married at the same time, a question that revealed my own assumption that married love meant being attached to one another. In answer to my question, the monk took a pen, clenched it in his hand, and palm down, extended his arm out in front of his body. "The pen is what I love," said the monk. "I hold on to what I love. If I open my hand," he said, slowly opening his hand, "I lose what I love because I have been holding on to it." The pen fell. He picked up the pen again and put it in his hand, wrapping his fingers around the pen, holding it tightly. This time, with palm up, he extended his arm out in front of his body. "Now, if I let go of the pen which I love," he said, slowly opening his hand, "it remains. This is how one loves without being attached."

Christianity also exclaims this paradox. "He who loses his life will find it, and he who finds his life will lose it" is one of those difficult sayings of Jesus. Parishioners have consistently asked me over the years what this saying of Jesus' means. Like the Buddhist monk's demonstration, it speaks to a spiritual reality. When we lose the outer indicators that define us, we often are forced to discover our inner identities, our unique and irreplaceable selves. Like the hand holding what we love, palm up, "He who loses his life"—opens his hand—"will find it" (the love remains), while "he who finds it"—holds on

to what he loves with palm down and opens his
hand—"will lose it."

  The desert is a place where one's identity is called into question and where it can emerge.
It isn't a nice place to be. It is lonely and without
comforts. It is scorching hot during the day and
bitter cold at night. The blackness and silence of
night is blacker and quieter than one can imagine.
The wilderness is a dangerous place—because it
lacks any protections—and a potential place of
introspection—because there are no distractions.
Step out of your car, and there are no gas stations, Internet, iPods, cell phones towers, TVs,
restaurants, mirrors, refrigerators, hotels, police
stations—nothing to stand in the way of facing
one's inner self.

  My mind wanders to the wilderness
scenes of the past, the place of birth of the three
monotheistic religions of the world, Judaism,
Christianity, and Islam. I think about the

Israelites wandering in the wilderness for forty years and ask, Why? I think of Jesus in the wilderness for forty days and ask, Why? The wilderness allows the shedding of externals and forces existential questions about the purpose and meaning of life. The wilderness is a threshold experience, leading us from one place to another.

After years of wandering, moaning and groaning, and learning new ways, the Israelites found the Promised Land; and after forty days of being tempted to lose sight of who he was, Jesus discovered his true self. Throughout history some individuals—the desert fathers, hermits, and persons of every religious persuasion—have gone into the desert voluntarily to undergo this process. Caregivers are thrown into it. Actually, the text in the Christian scriptures says that Jesus too was "thrown" into the wilderness after he was baptized by John. The Israelites, too, were not given a choice. Freedom required it, and that is true for our caregivers to be free too.

The desert, the place where everything we thought was important is left behind, the place of no mores, forces us to ask ourselves the question, Who am I?

An example that I find helpful comes from the story of Dietrich Bonhoeffer, the German Lutheran theologian and pastor who opposed Hitler in Nazi Germany during the Second World War and who was imprisoned in Flössenberg concentration camp for his part in the attempted assassination of Hitler. Hoping against hope that he would be released, but knowing on some level that he would be sentenced to death, he asked himself this question, Who am I?

The poem is very short and in three parts. In the first part, Bonhoeffer answers the question, Who am I? by stating what others say about him. We might say that this is the outer self that others see or the persona that we want others to see. They say he is calm and cheerful, and that even the guards regard him.

The second part is Bonhoeffer's answer to the question, *Who am I?* with his own self-assessment. Stripped of his freedom, his family, his church, his colleagues and friends, his home, his bed, his books, his work, and his future, he answers by listing his losses, his no mores, and his longings. Here he says he is restless, weary, and choking from his confinement, that he feels caged like a bird, longing for the sound of chirping birds, the sight of flowers, and colors and the deep desire for significant others that he is denied.

Finally, Bonhoeffer asks the question, *Who is accurate about who I am, the others or myself?* He wonders if he has deceived others and is a hypocrite. His ending is poignant. He discovers his core. What he may have said as theological and intellectual truth beforehand, he now can confess from his experience of being bereft *"Who am I? . . . Thou knowest, O God, I am Thine."*

When I was thirteen, I first encountered Bonhoeffer's poem in my church youth *group. It never made sense—why he, at thirty-nine, would write a poem with such a title—until I worked with the dying and caregivers and became involved with Holocaust studies.*

The wilderness is indeed a place of aloneness and a place without distractions. While this is not a nice time and we think we will never find our way out, we can tell the caregiver that the wilderness is a spiritual place that leads eventually, and with the right help and support, to a place of new identity. At this juncture, you as a professional caregiver have named the place of their confusion. It is a normal place to be, since they have been thrown out of their normal living place.

THE GENERAL
CONTRACTOR

IT is important to let caregivers know that society's expectation of them to do it all, their family's expectation for them to do it all, and even their own inner expectation that they should do it all, doesn't mean they have to do it alone. Eventually, every builder hires an architect, electrician, plumber, and painter, and when he has too many houses to build, he becomes the general contractor and gets all the help he can to get the jobs done.

In much the same way, caregivers need to discover, in this wilderness, their limitations—what they do well, what they don't do well, what they can't do at all, what they can and will learn, what they refuse to learn and do—and set out to get the help they need. Every caregiver must learn to let go of the idea that they have to do it all or meet someone else's expectations and must discover and be honest about their limitations and strengths. This is part of the discovery of the new self.

CAREGIVERS ALL

THE most difficult job is to be a caregiver. This needs to be acknowledged. It has been argued by the late Tom Kitwood, pioneer British researcher on dementia, that caring for persons with dementia takes us to the edge of our humanity and that only the most highly skilled and most creative persons can do this work.

German philosopher Martin Heidegger, claimed that care is the core of *being*, the essence of what it means to be a person; so Kitwood isn't the first to

raise and praise the phenomenon of care.
Care is the deeper development missing
in us as persons and in our society. We
see the greed, the attitude that I can make
as much as I want for myself, the iPod
versus the wePod world, the genocides
that continue with total disregard for
the other, the poor that are still among
us, because care is not valued highly, not
widely studied as a subject, and not culti-
vated intentionally.

In Holocaust studies, Samuel and
Pearl Oliner have studied why people
risked their lives to save others. They
have studied why people become hospice
volunteers. They have written about how
to develop a caring society.

As professional caregivers, it is
important for us to know what caring
means for us, to pass on to the caregivers in our charge the significance of what

they are being asked to do, and to travel with them on this very bumpy ride to a new and deeper sense of self. The spirit in us calls us to the care that is our core, the spiritual essence that connects each of us to the other.